AF406608

Keto Crock Pot Cookbook

Easy and Delicious Ketogenic Crock Pot
Recipes for Busy People

Jasmine King

The trademarks that are used are without any consent, and the publication of the trademark is without permission or backing by the trademark owner. All trademarks and brands within this book are for clarifying purposes only and are owned by the owners themselves, not affiliated with this document.

Table of Contents

CHAPTER FIVE

CHAPTER SIX

CHAPTER SEVEN

CHAPTER EIGHT

Ketogenic Soup Recipes 58

CHAPTER NINE

Ketogenic Snack Recipes 67

CHAPTER TEN

Ketogenic Dessert Recipes 72

CHAPTER ONE

Introduction of the Crock Pot: The Why and How

The Crock Pot is a slow cooker initially developed by the Naxon Corporation. When the company was purchased by The Rival Company the product was introduced with the Crock Pot name in 1971. Its popularity began in the 1970s and has increased over the decades.

While designs vary, a Crock Pot basically consists of a ceramic pot with a glass lid. The removable pot is placed inside a metal housing. The electric heating element is in the housing. As a Crock Pot is available in a number of sizes, you can find the perfect pot for every household.

Whether you have just purchased a Crock Pot or received one as a gift, it can make your life easier and more enjoyable.

Benefits of Using a Crock Pot

For most people, the most important benefit of a Crock Pot is convenience. Slow cooking takes up a lot less of your time and effort as compared to other methods of cooking where constant attention is a demand to be met. A full meal can be prepared in just a few minutes. When you use one pot to cook an entire meal, it is much easier than cooking with several pots and pans. People who have full-time jobs, attend school, or have other time-consuming responsibilities can start the meal in the morning and know it will be ready to eat when they come home.

Saving money is another benefit. You do not need to buy expensive cuts of your favorite meats because cheaper cuts will become tender, and the meat will never be tough or dry.

You will also save money because washing a Crock Pot uses much less water than washing many pots and pans.

Another feature of the Crock Pot to lust after has to be the flavor it creates. When the ingredients are cooked in this slow, simmering process in their own juices for hours, the amalgamation of flavors that is born is beyond anything frying, grilling, or even baking could achieve. The slow and steady cooking brings forth some of the unexpected flavors that add an extra dimension to slow-cooked meals.

How to Use a Crock Pot

It is always wise to read the instructions on a new appliance, but a slow cooker is quite simple.

First, consider safety. Make sure your outlet and wiring are in good condition so that the pot will not be a fire hazard. Always use the pot on a clean, dry surface, and never allow the cord to come in contact with water.

Exercise care when you open the pot and remove the food. As the liquid is very hot, it is easy to burn yourself if you are not careful.

Second, familiarize yourself with the settings. In general, the Low setting is used for foods you wish to simmer. The High setting is for foods you would normally fry, boil, or bake. High is the appropriate setting for meats, stews, desserts, and most recipes. The Warm setting is intended to keep food warm after it is cooked.

A third consideration is cleaning your Crock Pot. As the pots rarely require maintenance, all you need to do is carefully clean it after each use. While you can wash the pot and lid in the sink, never immerse the metal housing in water.

Tips for Crock Pot Cooking

A Crock Pot does not cause water to evaporate. If you are not using a recipe specially created for slow cookers, only add enough water to cover the food.

Regardless of the food you are cooking, water does not thicken. You can roll your meat in corn flour or seasoned flour before cooking. You can also make a paste of flour and water, and carefully add it to the simmering pot.

For the most flavorful dishes, try the low setting. Food will cook completely in the gentle heat.

If the dish you are making includes rice or pasta, add it shortly before the other ingredients have finished cooking. Texture and taste will be better.

Preparing your ingredients in advance helps a lot when you are running short on time. You could do your meal prep the night before; A common way to prep things up is to take all the ingredients that you have prepared and assemble it in the Crock Pot, cover it, and refrigerate overnight. The next day, remove it from the refrigerator; let it warm up to room temperature before starting the cooking process.

CHAPTER TWO

An Overview of the Ketogenic Diet

To describe it in simple terms, the ketogenic diet is a diet that is low in carbohydrates and high in fat. Traditionally, this diet was used as a way of controlling and treating certain diseases, but currently it is one of the most sought-after weight-loss diets. All around the world, people are raving about the benefits and the good changes it has brought about in their lives.

The ketogenic diet focuses on significantly reducing the body's carbohydrate intake and substituting it with fat. As a result, the body enters a metabolic state known as ketosis. During this stage, the body becomes extremely efficient at burning fat to make energy and converts the fat in the liver into ketones. The daily nutritional intake on a ketogenic diet is:

65–75% of calories from Fat,
25–30% from Protein, and
5–10% from Carbohydrates

Benefits of the Ketogenic Diet

Appetite Suppression
Since foods rich in fat tend to be satiating, their consumption in high amounts has the effect of reducing one's appetite.

Weight Loss
The most obvious benefit of this type of diet is weight loss. Even though you aren't restricting calories, your body will release the fat you don't need. The process of ketosis

ensures this. In the beginning there is rapid weight-loss because your body uses up its store of carbs. Then over a period of months, the weight loss reduces to a steady yet consistent pace. Weight loss comes with a long list of residual health benefits. You'll be at less risk for diabetes, high blood pressure, and strokes and heart attacks.

Maintaining Blood Sugar Levels

Carbohydrates are turned into sugars in our body. Following a keto diet helps in the regulation of our blood sugar levels. However, if you are pre-diabetic or suffer from diabetes, talk to your doctor first before starting the ketogenic diet.

Stable Energy Levels

Most people who switch to a ketogenic diet report how their energy levels remain high throughout the day. The reason is simple–fat is a readily available source of energy, which means the body is able to go for hours without food and not experience fluctuations in energy levels.

Treatment of Chronic Conditions

In addition to weight loss and a healthier lifestyle, the ketogenic diet is also used to treat illnesses and chronic conditions. It has been effective for people battling epilepsy and children who have suffered from prolonged and dangerous seizures.

What to Eat on a Ketogenic Diet?

If you're considering trying a low carbohydrate diet, you may envision yourself eating large amounts of meat. But there are many other foods to choose from. In fact, making sure you eat plenty of vegetables is very important to your overall health and weight loss goals.

Poultry and Meats: You are free to choose any kinds of meat including chicken, turkey, pork, beef, goat, lamb, and mutton. You can even eat the skin on the chicken!

Seafood and fish: You can eat any kind, but stick to the fattier kinds, such as mackerel, salmon, tuna, herring, and sardines.

Full-fat dairy products: Milk, yogurt, butter, cheeses, and sour cream.

Eggs

Nuts and seeds: Almonds, walnuts, flaxseeds, chia seeds, and pumpkin seeds.

Non-starchy vegetables: Cauliflower, asparagus, broccoli, zucchini, cabbage, tomatoes, squash, eggplants, leafy greens, Brussel sprouts, mushrooms, green bell peppers, and onions.

Fruits: Avocados are an absolute must. Berries can also be enjoyed often. Watch out for fruits that are rich sugar, such as apples, oranges, and mangoes.

Oils: Olive oil, flaxseed oil, avocado oil, coconut oil, and macadamia oil.

What to Avoid on a Ketogenic Diet?

Sugar: This is a keto dieter's worst enemy. You'll find sugar in most juices, soft drinks, cookies, candies, cakes, cereals, and ice creams.

Grains and products made from grains: Flour, pasta, baked goods, chips, wheat, and rice.

Starchy vegetables: Beans, potatoes, peas, lentils, parsnips, and corn.

Diet soda and fruit juices

Trans fats

If you are planning to follow the ketogenic diet, learning to prepare healthy ketogenic recipes is an important step towards achieving your goals. In this book, you will find 62 delicious ketogenic Crock Pot recipes for breakfast, poultry, meats, seafood, vegetables, soups, snacks, and dessert.

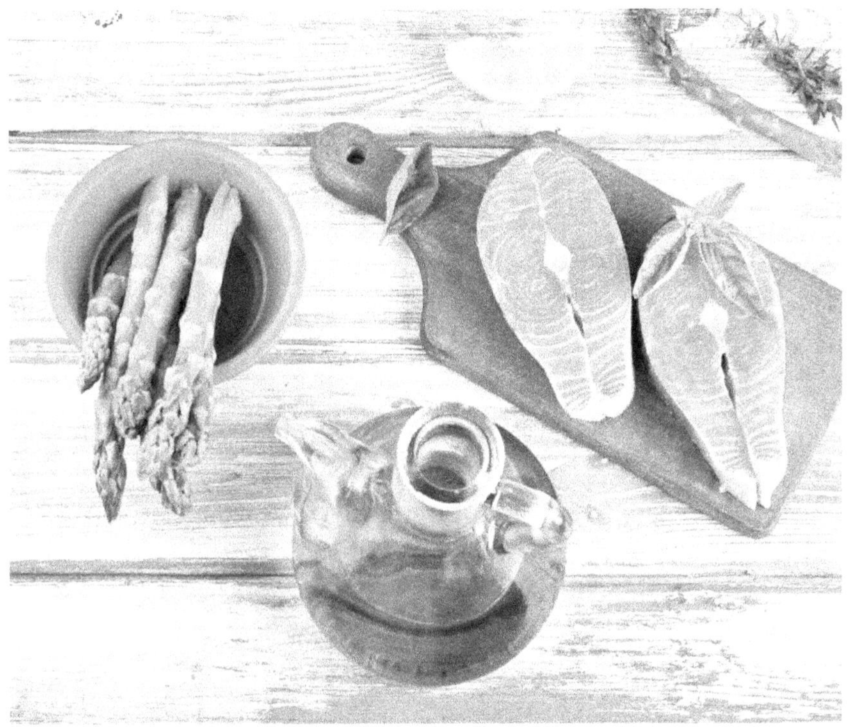

CHAPTER THREE

Ketogenic Breakfast Recipes

Breakfast Casserole

Serves: 8
Cooking Time: 7–8 hours
Ingredients:
12 large eggs
1 cup milk
Salt and pepper to taste
1 cup green bell pepper, chopped
2 ounces shallots, chopped
2 cups white mushrooms, chopped
16 large kale leaves, discard hard stem and ribs, finely chopped
6 large slices bacon, chopped
2 tablespoons butter, melted
2 cups Parmesan cheese, shredded

Directions:
1. In a bowl, add the eggs, milk, salt, and pepper, and beat until well combined.
2. Add bacon to a skillet. Place the skillet over medium heat. Cook until the bacon is crisp.
3. Stir in the green pepper, shallots, and mushrooms. Sauté for 1–2 minutes.
4. Add kale and stir. Turn off the heat.
5. Grease the inside of the Crock Pot with butter. Transfer the vegetable mixture into the pot.
6. Sprinkle with cheese. Add the egg mixture and stir to combine.

7. Close the lid. Set the Crock Pot on Low and cook for 7–8 hours or until set.

Nutritional Information (Per Serving)
Calories: 313; Fat: 22.2 g; Net Carbohydrates: 6.1 g; Protein: 22.9 g

Cauliflower Hash Brown Egg Cups

Serves: 6
Cooking Time: 6 hours
Ingredients:
1 head cauliflower, grated to rice like texture
¼ cup cheddar cheese or Mozzarella cheese
7 eggs
2 tablespoons Parmesan cheese, grated
Salt and pepper to taste
¼ teaspoon garlic powder

Directions:
1. Grease 6 muffin cups with cooking spray.

2. Lightly steam the cauliflower. Squeeze the cauliflower of excess moisture. Add into a bowl. Add 1 egg, cheese, salt, pepper, and garlic powder and mix well.

3. Divide into the 6 muffin cups. Press it into the cups making a well in each cup.

4. Place crumpled aluminum foil at the bottom of the Crock Pot (this step can be avoided if your pot is ceramic). Place the muffin molds inside the pot.

5. Close the lid. Set the pot on High and cook for 4 hours.

6. Open the lid and crack an egg in each muffin cup. Sprinkle with salt and pepper.

7. Cook on High for 2 hours or until the eggs are set as the way you like it cooked.

8. Cool for a while. Run a knife around the edges of the egg cups. Remove them carefully and serve.

Nutritional Information (Per Serving)
Calories: 87.7; Fat: 5.4 g; Net Carbohydrates: 2.2 g; Protein: 8 g

Spinach Quiche

Serves: 6
Cooking Time: 7–8 hours
Ingredients:
1 tablespoon butter, melted
1 onion, chopped
1 (10 ounces) package frozen spinach, thawed
5 eggs, beaten
1 cup milk
3 cups Muenster cheese, shredded
⅛ teaspoon red pepper flakes, crushed
Salt and pepper to taste

Directions:
1. Grease the inside of the Crock Pot with butter.
2. Add all ingredients and mix until well combined.
3. Close the lid, set the Crock Pot on Low, and cook for 7–8 hours.
4. Cut into 6 wedges of equal size and serve.

Nutritional Information (Per Serving)
Calories: 296; Fat: 22.7 g; Net Carbohydrates: 2.9 g; Protein: 19.4 g

Easy Frittata

Serves: 8
Cooking Time: 8–9 hours
Ingredients:
12 large eggs, beaten
1 cup milk
1½ cups artichoke hearts, chopped
½ cup green bell pepper, chopped
Salt and pepper to taste
1 tomato, deseeded, chopped
½ cup green onion, chopped
½ cup cheddar cheese, grated

Directions:
1. Spray the bottom of the Crock Pot with cooking spray.

2. Add all the ingredients except cheese into a bowl and mix well. Pour into the Crock Pot.

3. Close the lid. Set the pot on Low and cook for 8–9 hours or until desired doneness of eggs.

4. Sprinkle cheese on top. Cover and let it sit for a few minutes.

5. Slice into 8 wedges and serve.

Nutritional Information (Per Serving)
Calories:141; Fat: 9 g; Net Carbohydrate: 3.1 g; Protein: 12 g

Veggie Omelet

Serves: 2
Cooking Time: 2–3 hours
Ingredients:

3 eggs
¼ cup milk
A pinch chili powder
1 clove garlic, minced
Salt and pepper to taste
1 tablespoon butter, melted
½ green bell pepper, chopped
½ cup broccoli florets
½ small yellow onion, chopped
1 cup cheddar cheese, grated
Chopped tomatoes, onions, and parsley as topping

Directions:

1. In a bowl, add eggs, milk, chili powder, garlic, salt, and pepper, and beat until well combined.

2. Grease the Crock Pot with butter. In the bottom of the Crock Pot, mix together the bell pepper, broccoli, and onion.

3. Pour egg mixture on top, and gently stir to combine.

4. Set the Crock Pot on High. Cover and cook for about 2–3 hours or until desired doneness of eggs.

5. When done, sprinkle cheese on it. Cover and let it sit for a few minutes.

6. Carefully transfer the omelet onto a plate. Cut into 2 and serve with toppings.

Nutritional Information (Per Serving)
Calories: 302; Fat: 22.5 g; Net Carbohydrates: 7 g; Protein: 17.7 g

Creamy Keto Hot Cocoa

Serves: 4
Cooking Time: 1½ hour
Ingredients:
3 cups coconut milk, unsweetened
4 tablespoons cocoa powder
1 teaspoon vanilla extract
2 tablespoons Swerve
4 tablespoons heavy whipping cream
2 teaspoons instant coffee
1 teaspoon ground cinnamon

Directions:
1. Add milk and cream into the Crock Pot.
2. Close the lid, set the pot on High, and cook for 1½ hours.
3. Add rest of the ingredients during the last 30 minutes of cook time. Whisk well.
4. Pour into mugs and serve.

Nutritional Information (Per Serving)
Calories:104; Fat: 9.6 g; Net Carbohydrates: 6.1 g; Protein: 1.5 g

Sweet Sausage and Peppers

Serves: 6
Cooking Time: 3 hours 10 minutes
Ingredients:
12 ounces breakfast sausage, cut into pieces
1 cup red onion, sliced
2 cups mushrooms, sliced
2 cups green bell pepper
1 teaspoon olive oil
¼ cup water
2 teaspoons fresh parsley
2 teaspoons fresh tarragon

Directions:

1. Brown your sausage in a skillet for 5 minutes, and then stir the onion in the same skillet with the olive oil until it starts to soften.

2. Combine the sausage, onion, and mushrooms in the Crock Pot. Pour the water over the top.

3. Cover the Crock Pot, and let it cook on High for 2 hours.

4. Stir in the bell pepper and allow it to cook for one more hour.

5. Sprinkle with parsley and tarragon before serving.

Nutritional Information (Per Serving)
Calories: 243; Fat: 18.6 g; Net Carbohydrates: 5.1 g; Protein: 12.6 g

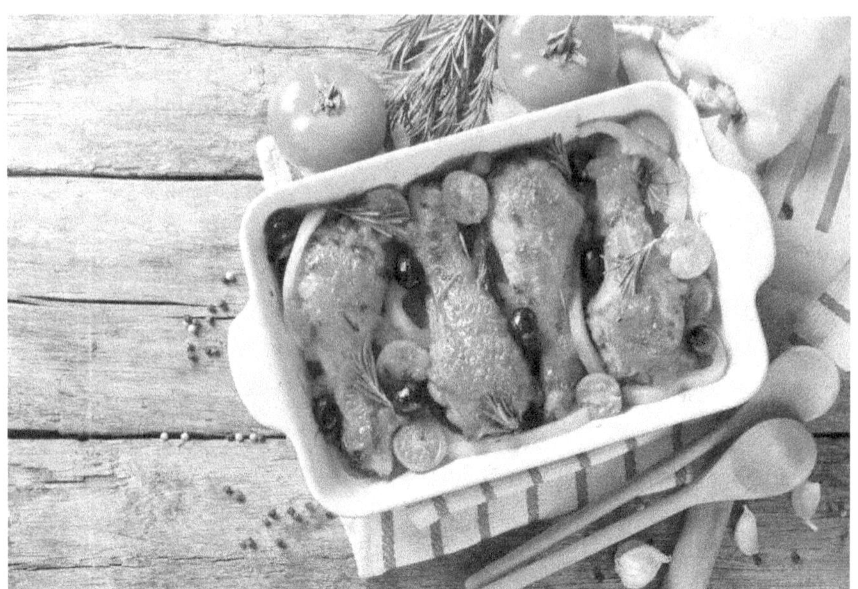

CHAPTER FOUR

Ketogenic Poultry Recipes

Ranch Chicken

Serves: 3
Cooking Time: 4 hours 45 minutes
Ingredients:
For ranch seasoning mix:
½ tablespoon dried parsley
¾ teaspoon dried dill
¼ teaspoon dried onion
¼ teaspoon salt
1 teaspoon dried chives
¼ teaspoon paprika
¼ teaspoon garlic powder
Freshly ground pepper to taste

For ranch chicken:
3 chicken breast halves, skinless, boneless
¾ teaspoon steak seasoning
2 teaspoons ranch seasoning mix (given above)
½ cup chicken broth
2 small shallots, sliced
6 slices bacon
3 cups broccoli florets
¼ cup keto friendly mayonnaise
Salt to taste
1½ tablespoons red wine vinegar

Directions:
1. Mix together all the ingredients of ranch seasoning in a small jar. Use 2 teaspoons of it.

2. Place chicken in the Crock Pot. Season the chicken with ranch seasoning and steak seasoning. Add the broth and place shallots on top.

3. Close the lid. Set the pot on Low and cook for 3 hours.

4. Add broccoli and cook for 45 minutes.

5. Meanwhile, cook the bacon in a skillet until crisp. Crumble the bacon when cooled.

6. When the chicken is done, shred it and add it back into the pot. Add vinegar, salt, bacon, and mayonnaise and mix well.

7. Serve warm.

Nutritional Information (Per Serving)
Calories: 424; Fat: 23.3 g; Net Carbohydrates: 7.2 g; Protein: 39.1 g

Chicken Breasts with Creamy Sauce

Serves: 4
Cooking Time: 4–5 hours
Ingredients:
4 (6 ounces) chicken breasts
5 tablespoons butter, melted
2 small onions, chopped
3 garlic cloves, minced
1 teaspoon dried tarragon, crushed
8 ounces cream cheese, softened
1 cup chicken broth
2 tablespoons lemon juice
½ cup heavy cream
1½ teaspoons Herbes de Provence
Salt and pepper to taste

Directions:
1. Place the chicken in the Crock Pot, season with salt and pepper.

2. Add the rest ingredients to the pot and mix well.

3. Close the lid, set the pot on Low, and cook for 4–5 hours.

4. Serve warm.

Nutritional Information (Per Serving)
Calories: 599; Fat: 44.4 g; Net Carbohydrates: 6 g; Protein: 42.2 g

Buffalo Chicken

Serves: 3
Cooking Time: 7 hours
Ingredients:
3 chicken breasts
2 teaspoons ranch seasoning mix
½ cup hot sauce
1½ tablespoons butter

Directions:
1. Place chicken in the Crock Pot. Drizzle hot sauce over it. Season with ranch seasoning.

2. Close the lid. Set the pot on Low and cook for 6 hours.

3. Remove the chicken with a slotted spoon. Shred the chicken and add it back into the pot.

4. Add butter and cook without the lid on Low for an hour.

Nutritional Information (Per Serving)
Calories: 336; Fat: 16.7 g; Net Carbohydrates: 0.6 g; Protein: 42.5 g

Pizza Chicken

Serves: 4
Cooking Time: 5–6 hours
Ingredients:
1¼ pounds chicken breast, chopped
10 ounces keto friendly pizza sauce
½ teaspoon garlic powder
½ teaspoon dried oregano
2 tablespoons olive oil
1 green pepper, sliced
¼ cup mushrooms, sliced
½ ounce pepperoni slices
½ cup pizza cheese
1 small onion, sliced

Directions:
1. Grease the inside of the Crock Pot with cooking spray.

2. Place chicken at the bottom of the Crock Pot. Spread pizza sauce over it. Sprinkle with garlic powder, oregano, and olive oil.

3. Layer with vegetables, mushrooms, pepperoni slices, and cheese.

4. Close the lid, set the pot on High, and cook for 5–6 hours.

Nutritional Information (Per Serving)
Calories: 398; Fat: 19.9 g; Net Carbohydrates: 8.6 g; Protein: 42.2 g

Chicken Stew

Serves: 2
Cooking Time: 6–8 hours
Ingredients:
1 cup chicken stock
2 cups chicken, skinless, boneless, chopped into chunks
1 stalk celery, chopped
3 cloves garlic, minced
¼ cup onion, chopped
¼ teaspoon dried rosemary
¼ teaspoon dried oregano
¼ teaspoon dried thyme
1 tablespoon olive oil
½ cup fresh spinach, chopped
Salt and pepper to taste
½ cup heavy cream
⅛ teaspoon xanthan gum

Directions:

1. Add celery, chicken, stock, garlic, onion, herbs, and olive oil into the Crock Pot and stir.

2. Close the lid, set the pot on Low and cook for 6–8 hours.

3. Add spinach, salt, pepper, and cream.

4. Sprinkle some xanthan gum to get the desired thickness. Whisk well.

5. Heat thoroughly. Ladle into bowls and serve.

Nutritional Information (Per Serving)
Calories: 419; Fat: 22.8 g; Net Carbohydrates: 7.9 g; Protein: 42.8 g

Low Carb Turkey Chili

Serves: 6
Cooking Time: 7 hours
Ingredients:
2 tablespoons olive oil
4 cloves garlic, minced
1 green bell pepper, chopped
1 pound ground turkey
7½ ounces canned diced tomatoes
7½ ounces canned pumpkin puree
1 tablespoon chili powder
½ teaspoon ground cumin
½ teaspoon onion powder
3 ounces tomato paste
¾ cup chicken broth
1 teaspoon ground cinnamon
½ teaspoon sea salt or to taste
Freshly ground pepper to taste

Directions:
1. Place a skillet with oil over medium high heat. Add pepper and garlic. Sauté for a couple of minutes until garlic turns aromatic.
2. Add ground turkey. Sauté until the meat is not pink anymore.
3. Transfer into the Crock Pot.
4. Add rest of the ingredients and mix well.
5. Close the lid. Set the pot on Low and cook for 7 hours.
6. Ladle into bowls and serve.

Nutritional Information (Per Serving)
Calories: 238; Fat: 13.7 g; Net Carbohydrates: 7.4 g; Protein: 23.2 g

Bacon Wrapped Turkey Breast with Tomatoes

Serves: 8
Cooking Time: 4 hours
Ingredients:
2 pounds turkey breast, chopped
6 tomatoes, peeled and chopped
2 bay leaves
16 ounces bacon slices, thinly cut
¼ teaspoon garlic powder
Salt and pepper to taste

Directions:
1. Take the bacon slices and wrap it around the turkey.
2. Add rest of the ingredients into the Crock Pot and stir.
3. Place the turkey in the pot.
4. Close the lid. Set the pot on High and cook for 4 hours.
5. Discard bay leaves. Slice the turkey and serve with the cooked sauce.

Nutritional Information (Per Serving)
Calories: 369; Fat: 24.7 g; Net Carbohydrates: 4 g; Protein: 32.1 g

Slow Cooked Turkey Breast

Serves: 6
Cooking Time: 8 hours
Ingredients:
Salt and pepper to taste
2½ pounds bone-in skin-on turkey breast
2 tablespoons olive oil
3 tablespoons Stubbs' chicken spice rub mixture
½ cup chicken broth

Directions:
1. Sprinkle salt and pepper over the turkey.
2. Place the turkey in the Crock Pot. Rub the olive oil and spice rub over it.
3. Add the broth and close the lid.
4. Set the pot on High and cook for 1 hour and then on Low for 7 hours.

Nutritional Information (Per Serving)
Calories: 336; Fat: 17.9 g; Net Carbohydrates: 0; Protein: 41 g

CHAPTER FIVE

Ketogenic Meat Recipes

Beef Curry

Serves: 4
Cooking Time: 4 hours
Ingredients:

1¼ pounds chuck roast

1 cup water

3 tablespoons coconut milk powder

1½ tablespoons Thai red curry paste

3 pods cardamom, cracked

½ tablespoon dried onion flakes

½ tablespoon swerve

½ tablespoon ground coriander

A pinch ground nutmeg

1 tablespoon Thai fish sauce

1 tablespoon dried or fresh Thai red chilies

½ tablespoon ground cumin

A pinch ground cloves

½ tablespoon ground ginger

To serve:

1 tablespoon coconut milk powder

1 tablespoon swerve

2 tablespoons cashew, chopped

½ tablespoon Thai red curry paste

A pinch xanthan gum (optional)

A handful fresh cilantro, chopped

Directions:

1. Add all the ingredients into the Crock Pot and stir.

2. Close the lid. Set the pot on High and cook for 4 hours.

3. Remove the meat with a slotted spoon and place in a bowl. Chop or break into smaller pieces.

4. Add all the serving ingredients except cilantro into the Crock Pot and mix.

5. Add the meat back into the pot. Mix well.

6. Garnish with cilantro and serve.

Nutritional Information (Per Serving)
Calories: 351; Fat: 22.8 g; Net Carbohydrates: 5.2 g; Protein: 26 g

Hungarian Goulash

Serves: 4
Cooking Time: 8 hours
Ingredients:
1 tablespoon butter
1 tablespoon Hungarian paprika
1 pound beef stew meat, cubed
¼ teaspoon pepper powder or to taste
½ teaspoon salt or to taste
¼ teaspoon caraway seeds
1 bell pepper of any color, chopped
7½ ounces canned diced tomatoes
1 bay leaf
½ cup onion, chopped
1 clove garlic, sliced
1 cup daikon radish, cubed
1 stalk celery, chopped
¾ cup beef broth

Directions:
1. Place a skillet with butter over medium heat. When it melts, add onions and sauté until translucent.

2. Add garlic and sauté for a few seconds until fragrant. Add paprika and sauté for 5–8 seconds.

3. Add beef and cook until brown. Add salt, pepper and caraway seeds and stir. Transfer into the Crock Pot.

4. Add rest of the ingredients and stir.

5. Close the lid. Set the pot on Low and cook for 8 hours or on High for 4 hours.

6. You can top with zucchini noodles to complete a meal.

Nutritional Information (Per Serving, without noodles)
Calories: 345; Fat: 23.9 g; Net Carbohydrates: 8.3 g; Protein: 23.8 g

Mississippi Roast

Serves: 4
Cooking Time: 4 hours
Ingredients:
2 pounds beef chuck roast
½ tablespoon dried parsley
½ tablespoon garlic powder
½ tablespoon dried dill
½ tablespoon dried chives
½ tablespoon onion powder
Salt and pepper to taste
8 ounces jarred deli-sliced pepperoncini's, retain the brine
4 tablespoons butter
1 tablespoon better than beef bouillon

Directions:
1. Add meat into the Crock Pot. Place pepperoncini's over it. Pour ½ cup of retained brine into the pot. Add rest of the ingredients except butter and stir.

2. Place butter on top of the meat.

3. Close the lid. Set the pot on High and cook for 4 hours or until meat comes off the bone.

4. Remove the meat with a slotted spoon and place in a bowl. Shred with a pair of forks and add it back into the pot.

5. Stir and serve.

Nutritional Information (Per Serving)
Calories: 435; Fat: 31.6 g; Net Carbohydrates: 4.3 g; Protein: 33.2 g

Beef and Cabbage Stew

Serves: 6
Cooking Time: 9 hours
Ingredient:
2 pounds beef stew meat, trimmed and cubed
Salt and pepper to taste
5 cups green cabbage, chopped
1 large onion, chopped
4 garlic cloves, minced
4 fresh tomatoes, chopped finely
1 cup beef broth
¼ cup fresh parsley, chopped

Directions:
1. Season the beef generously with salt and pepper.
2. In the bottom of a large Crock Pot, place the cabbage, onion, and garlic.
4. Top with beef, followed by tomatoes. Pour broth evenly on top and stir gently to combine.
5. Set the Crock Pot on Low. Cover and cook for about 9 hours.
6. Serve with a garnish of fresh parsley.

Nutritional Information (Per Serving)
Calories: 452; Fat: 31.8 g; Net Carbohydrates: 7.8 g; Protein: 29.7 g

Barbecue Beef Stew

Serves: 3
Cooking Time: 7 hours 30 minutes
Ingredients:
For barbecue sauce:
3½ ounces tomato paste
½ teaspoon salt
½ teaspoon smoked paprika
1 tablespoon erythritol or stevia
6 tablespoons balsamic vinegar
½ teaspoon garlic powder
¼ teaspoon black pepper

For stew:
1 pound beef stew meat, boneless, cubed
¼ teaspoon pepper
½ teaspoon arrowroot starch mixed with 1 tablespoon water
½ teaspoon salt
½ tablespoon olive oil

Directions:
1. Add all the ingredients of barbecue sauce in a bowl and whisk well.
2. Sprinkle salt and pepper over beef.
3. Place a skillet with oil over medium heat. Add beef and cook until brown on all the sides. Transfer into the Crock Pot.
4. Pour sauce into the pot and mix well.
5. Cover, set the pot on Low, and cook for 7 hours.
6. Add arrowroot starch mixture and stir. Cook on High for 20–30 minutes.
7. Serve warm.

Low Carb Meatloaf

Serves: 8
Cooking Time: 5–6 hours
Ingredients:
For meatloaf:
3 pounds ground beef
3 teaspoons salt
¾ cup cheddar cheese, shredded
¾ cup Parmesan cheese, shredded
3 large eggs
1 yellow onion, diced
1½ teaspoons garlic powder

To serve: Optional
Parmesan or Swiss cheese
Keto friendly ketchup

Directions:
1. Take a loaf pan that fits well inside the Crock Pot. Spray with cooking spray.

2. Add all the ingredients of meatloaf into a bowl and mix using your hands.

3. Transfer into the prepared loaf pan.

4. Place 2 long (folded lengthwise) strips of foil in a crisscross manner in the Crock Pot. Place the loaf pan over the foil.

5. Close the lid. Set the pot on High and cook for 5–6 hours or the internal temperature of the meat when checked with a cooking thermometer shows 160° F.

6. If you want to use Swiss cheese, place it now on the hot meatloaf.

7. Slice into 12 equal slices and serve with keto friendly ketchup if desired.

Nutritional Information (Per Serving)
Calories: 414; Fat: 27 g; Net Carbohydrates: 2 g; Protein: 38.8 g

Ketogenic Pizza

Serves: 8
Cooking Time: 4 hours
Ingredients:
1 28-ounce can whole tomatoes
1 6-ounce can tomato paste
1 pound Italian sausage
½ stick pepperoni, sliced
1 cup black olives
1 red onion, sliced
1 cup mushrooms, chopped
1 green bell pepper, chopped
3 cloves garlic, minced
½ cup water
4 sprigs thyme, chopped
6 fresh basil leaves, chopped

Directions:

1. Remove sausage from casing and cook in a skillet until brown.

2. Place the sausage and all the other ingredients into the Crock Pot, and stir until everything is combined.

3. Cook on High for 4 hours.

4. Feel free to customize this recipe to add all your favorite pizza toppings.

Nutritional Information (Per Serving)
Calories: 569; Fat: 51.3 g; Net Carbohydrates: 9.2 g; Protein: 16.7 g

Spicy Beef Brisket

Serves: 12
Cooking Time: 6–8 hours
Ingredients:
1 tablespoon olive oil
1 large white onion, sliced
3 garlic cloves, minced
1 (4 pounds) beef brisket
½ teaspoon red pepper flakes, crushed
½ teaspoon paprika
½ teaspoon ground cumin
¼ teaspoon ground cinnamon
Salt and pepper to taste
½ cup beef broth

Directions:
1. In a large Crock Pot, add all ingredients, and mix well.
2. Set the Crock Pot on Low. Cover and cook for 6–8 hours.
3. Uncover the Crock Pot, and transfer the brisket onto a cutting board.
4. Set aside for about 10 minutes before slicing.
5. With a sharp knife, cut into desired slices.
6. Serve with fresh green salad.

Nutritional Information (Per Serving)
Calories: 300; Fat: 10.7 g; Net Carbohydrates: 1.6 g; Protein: 46.3 g

Hungarian Paprika Pork

Serves: 4
Cooking Time: 8 hours
Ingredients:
1¼ pounds pork tenderloin
2 tablespoons butter, melt
2 cloves garlic, minced
½ tablespoon paprika
½ tablespoon Worcestershire sauce
2 tablespoons chicken broth
A handful fresh thyme, chopped
½ cup onion, chopped
1 small red bell pepper, diced
¼ teaspoon ground caraway
4 teaspoons red wine vinegar
2 tablespoons tomato paste
½ cup sour cream
Salt and pepper to taste

Directions:
1. Sprinkle salt and pepper over the pork, brush with butter, and place in the Crock Pot.

2. Add onion, garlic, pepper, and thyme.

3. Add rest of the ingredients except sour cream into a bowl. Mix well and pour over the pork.

4. Close the lid. Set the pot on Low and cook for 8 hours.

5. Remove the pork with a slotted spoon and place on your cutting board. When cool enough to handle, shred the pork with a pair of forks.

6. Add the pork back into the pot. Stir well. Cook for 10 minutes without the lid.

7. Add sour cream. Stir and serve.

Crock Pot Pork

Serves: 3
Cooking Time: 8 hours
Ingredients:
1¼ pounds pork tenderloin
1 clove garlic, minced
1 cup chicken broth
1 teaspoon ground cumin
½ teaspoon paprika
1 tablespoons olive oil
Salt and pepper to taste
1 tablespoon Worcestershire sauce

Directions:
1. Add all the ingredients into the Crock Pot.
2. Close the lid. Set the pot on Low and cook for 8 hours or on High for 4 hours.
3. When done, shred or slice the pork and serve topped with the liquid in the pot.

Nutritional Information (Per Serving)
Calories: 263; Fat: 12 g; Net Carbohydrates: 1.9 g; Protein: 33 g

Low Carb Pork Chops with Spice Rub

Serves: 4
Cooking Time: 4 hours
Ingredients:
1 pound pork chops
½ tablespoons dried rosemary
½ tablespoon curry powder
½ tablespoon fennel seeds
½ teaspoon salt
½ tablespoon dried thyme
½ tablespoon fresh chives, chopped
½ tablespoon ground cumin
2 tablespoons olive oil
½ cup beef broth

Directions:
1. Pour half the oil into the Crock Pot.
2. In a bowl, mix together rest of the ingredients except the pork chops and broth, and rub it all over the chops.
3. Add broth to the pot, place the chops in it, and close the lid.
4. Set the pot on High and cook for 4 hours.

Nutritional Information (Per Serving)
Calories: 247; Fat: 15 g; Net Carbohydrates: 1 g; Protein: 24 g

Lamb Barbacoa

Serves: 6
Cooking Time: 6 hours
Ingredients:
2¼ pounds leg of lamb, boneless
1 tablespoon salt
½ tablespoon ground cumin
2 tablespoons dried mustard
1 tablespoon paprika
½ teaspoon chipotle powder
½ tablespoon dried oregano
½ cup water

Directions:
1. Sprinkle mustard over the lamb. Mix together all the spices in a bowl and sprinkle over the lamb. Refrigerate for 6–8 hours if possible.

2. Place lamb in the Crock Pot. Add the water.

3. Close the lid. Set the pot on High and cook for 6 hours.

4. Remove the lamb with a slotted spoon and place on your cutting board. When cool enough to handle, shred with a pair of forks. Add lamb back into the pot.

5. Mix well and serve.

Nutritional Information (Per Serving)
Calories: 492; Fat: 35.8 g; Net Carbohydrates: 1.2 g; Protein: 37.5 g

Mustard Rosemary Lamb

Serves: 8
Cooking Time: 8 hours
Ingredients:
3 pounds leg of lamb
3 tablespoons whole grain mustard
6 sprigs thyme
1¼ teaspoons dried rosemary
Salt and pepper to taste
6 tablespoons olive oil
½ cup beef broth
A handful fresh mint leaves
1½ teaspoons garlic, minced

Directions:
1. Score the lamb at 4–5 places. Place garlic and rosemary in the slits.

2. Place in the Crock Pot. Rub oil over it. Sprinkle mustard, salt, and pepper over it and rub it well.

3. Add the broth and close the lid.

4. Set the pot on Low and cook for 8 hours. Add thyme and mint during the last hour of cooking.

Nutritional Information (Per Serving)
Calories: 490; Fat: 39.4 g; Net Carbohydrate: 1.2 g; Protein: 30.4 g

Slow Cooked Lamb Leg

Serves: 2
Cooking Time: 8 hours
Ingredients:
2 pounds lamb leg
1 sprig fresh rosemary
Salt to taste
3 tablespoons balsamic vinegar
2 cloves garlic, minced
1 head lettuce
1 cup water

Directions:
1. Place lamb in the Crock Pot.

2. Add rest of the ingredients except lettuce into a bowl and mix well. Pour over the lamb.

3. Close the lid. Set the pot on Low and cook for 8 hours or on High for 4 hours.

4. Remove the lamb with a slotted spoon and place on your cutting board. When cool enough to handle, shred the lamb with a pair of forks.

5. Add the lamb back into the pot. Stir well. Cook for 10 minutes without the lid.

6. Place the lettuce leaves on a serving platter. Spoon the lamb on it and serve.

Nutritional Information (Per Serving)
Calories: 574; Fat: 38.4 g; Net Carbohydrates: 7.5 g; Protein: 46.5 g

CHAPTER SIX

Ketogenic Seafood Recipes

Poached Salmon

Serves: 8
Cooking Time: 1½ hours
Ingredients:
4 cups water
2 bay leaves
2 teaspoons black peppercorns
8 salmon fillets
4 sprigs of rosemary
2 cloves garlic, minced
2 teaspoons kosher salt
Freshly ground pepper and salt to taste
2 lemons, thinly sliced

To serve:
Lemon wedges
Olive oil
Coarse sea salt

Directions:
1. Add water, bay leaves, black peppercorns, rosemary, and garlic into the pot.

2. Close the lid. Set the pot on High and cook for 30 minutes.

3. Sprinkle salt and pepper over the salmon and place in the Crock Pot.

4. Set the pot on High and cook for 1 hour. Keep a check on the salmon after 45 minutes of cooking. Cook until done.

5. Remove the salmon with a slotted spoon and place on a serving platter.

6. Sprinkle with sea salt and drizzle oil and serve with lemon wedges.

Nutritional Information (Per Serving)
Calories: 504; Fat: 30.5 g; Net Carbohydrates: 1.5 g; Protein: 46.5 g

Seafood Stew

Serves: 6
Cooking Time: 6 hours 45 minutes
Ingredients:
4 tablespoons butter, melted
1 medium onion, chopped
2 garlic cloves, minced
1 serrano pepper, chopped
¼ teaspoon red pepper flakes, crushed
¾ pound fresh tomatoes, chopped
1½ cups water
1 pound red snapper fillets, cubed
½ pound shrimp, peeled and deveined
¼ pound squid, cleaned and cut into rings
¼ pound scallops
¼ pound mussels
2 tablespoons fresh lime juice
½ cup of chopped fresh basil
Salt and pepper to taste
⅓ cup mayonnaise

Directions:

1. Place all ingredients, except for the seafood and mayonnaise, in the Crock Pot and stir.

2. Close the lid and cook on Low for 6 hours.

3. Add the seafood and set the pot on High.

4. Cook for another 45 minutes, but check on the seafood after 30 minutes. You don't want to overcook.

5. Serve hot with a topping of mayonnaise.

Nutritional Information (Per Serving)
Calories: 333; Fat: 15 g; Net Carbohydrates: 8.8 g; Protein: 38 g

Indonesian Fish

Serves: 6
Cooking Time: 5 hours
Ingredients:
1 large onion, sliced
4 tablespoons fresh lime juice
3 pounds fish steak (use halibut or swordfish)
3 tablespoons soy sauce
Salt to taste
Crushed red pepper flakes to taste
2 tablespoons olive oil
½ teaspoon ground pepper
1 teaspoon ground coriander

Directions:
1. Add half the onions, soy sauce, lime juice, coriander, crushed red pepper, salt, pepper, and olive oil into a bowl and mix well. Place the fish pieces in it. Turn the fish so that it is well coated.

2. Sprinkle the rest of the onions over the fish. Cover the bowl with cling wrap.

3. Place the bowl in the refrigerator for 3–4 hours.

4. Transfer the ingredients into the Crock Pot.

5. Close the lid. Set the pot on High and cook for 2 hours.

6. Transfer on to a serving platter. Pour the cooking liquid over the fish and serve.

Nutritional Information (Per Serving)
Calories: 310; Fat: 13.3 g; Net Carbohydrates: 3.0 g; Protein: 48.8 g

Fish Curry

Serves: 8
Cooking Time: 4 hours
Ingredients:
2 tablespoons ginger, minced
3 tablespoons curry powder
3 tablespoons olive oil
1 teaspoon ground cinnamon
4 cloves garlic, minced
1 teaspoon turmeric powder
1 teaspoon chili powder
1 bell pepper, finely chopped
1 chili pepper, chopped
2 tomatoes, chopped
1 cup water
3 pounds tilapia, cubed

Directions:

1. Add all the ingredients except tilapia into the Crock Pot and stir.

2. Close the lid. Set the pot on Low and cook for 4 hours. Add tilapia during the last 45 minutes of cook time.

3. Stir and serve.

Nutritional Information (Per Serving)
Calories: 212; Fat: 15.9 g; Net Carbohydrates: 3.9 g; Protein: 32.6 g

Spicy Seafood Stew

Serves: 2
Cooking Time: 6 hours
Ingredients:
½ cup chicken broth
1 small bell pepper, chopped
1 small onion, chopped
7 ounces canned diced tomatoes
1 clove garlic, minced
4 ounces tomato sauce
½ teaspoon Splenda
Hot pepper sauce to taste
½ cup water
1 bay leaf
2 tablespoons olive oil
¼ teaspoon Cajun seasoning
1½ teaspoons dried thyme
3 ounces shrimp, peeled, deveined
4 ounces fish fillets, skinless, cut into 1 inch pieces
A handful fresh parsley, chopped, to garnish

Directions:
1. Add all the ingredients except seafood to the Crock Pot. Mix well.

2. Close the lid. Set the pot on Low and cook for 6 hours or on High for 3 hours.

3. Add the seafood during the last 30 minutes of cooking and stir.

4. Stir occasionally while it is cooking.

5. Ladle into soup bowls. Garnish with parsley and serve.

Nutritional Information (Per Serving)
Calories: 337; Fat: 22.2 g; Net Carbohydrates: 14.5 g; Protein: 20.1 g

Lemon Pepper Tilapia with Asparagus

Serves: 8
Cooking Time: 3 hours
Ingredients:
8 tilapia fillets
20 asparagus spears, chopped
8 teaspoons lemon pepper seasoning or to taste
4 tablespoons butter
½ cup lemon juice

Directions:
1. Take 8 foils. Lay the fillets in the middle of the foil. Sprinkle 1 teaspoon lemon pepper seasoning over it.

2. Place ½ tablespoon of butter on each of the fillets. Divide and place asparagus over the fish.

3. Wrap foil all around the fish. Seal it well.

4. Place the packets in the Crock Pot. It can be overlapped while placing it.

5. Close lid. Set the pot on High and cook for 2 hours if thawed and for 3 hours if frozen.

Nutritional Information (Per Serving)
Calories: 208; Fat: 9 g; Net Carbohydrates: 1.7 g; Protein: 33.3 g

Shrimp Scampi

Serves: 8
Cooking Time: 2–3 hours
Ingredients:
½ cup chicken broth
4 tablespoons olive oil
2 tablespoons garlic, minced
2 tablespoons lemon juice
2 pounds raw shrimp, peeled and deveined
4 tablespoons butter
¼ cup parsley, finely chopped + extra to garnish
Salt and pepper to taste
1 teaspoon red pepper flakes
Parmesan cheese, grated to garnish

Directions:
1. Add all the ingredients except Parmesan cheese into the Crock Pot and stir.

2. Close the lid. Set the pot on Low and cook for 2–3 hours or on High for 1–1 ½ hours.

3. Garnish with Parmesan and serve.

Nutritional Information (Per Serving)
Calories: 256; Fat: 14.7 g; Net Carbohydrates: 2.1 g; Protein: 23.3 g

CHAPTER SEVEN

Ketogenic Vegetable Recipes

Stuffed Mushrooms

Serves: 2
Cooking Time: 3 hours
Ingredients:
1 pound mushrooms
½ cup chicken broth
8 ounces Boursin cheese
Paprika to garnish

Directions:
1. Remove the stems from the mushrooms, and reserve them for another use.

2. Fill all the mushrooms with Boursin cheese, and place them at the bottom of the Crock Pot.

3. Pour some chicken broth around the mushrooms to fill the bottom of the pot. Sprinkle with paprika.

4. Close the lid. Set the pot on High and cook for 2–3 hours.

5. Serve hot.

Nutritional Information (Per Serving)
Calories: 512; Fat: 50.1 g; Net Carbohydrates: 9.1 g; Protein: 15.9 g

Zucchini Gratin

Serves: 4
Cooking Time: 3 hours
Ingredients:
2 cups zucchini slices
Salt and pepper to taste
1 tablespoon butter, melted
¼ cup heavy whipping cream
½ small onion, thinly sliced
¾ cup pepper Jack cheese, shredded
¼ teaspoon garlic powder

Directions:
1. Grease the inside of the Crock Pot with a little oil butter.

2. Place onion slices at the bottom of the pot. Layer with zucchini slices followed by cheese.

3. Mix together the rest of the ingredients in a bowl and pour over the cheese layer.

4. Close the lid. Set the pot on High and cook for 2–3 hours or until zucchini is tender.

5. Let it sit for a while before serving. Slice into 4 equal portions and serve.

Nutritional Information (Per Serving)
Calories: 230; Fat: 20.1 g; Net Carbohydrates: 3 g; Protein: 8 g

Cheesy Cauliflower Puree

Serves: 8
Cooking Time: 3 hours
Ingredients:
4 cups cauliflower florets
½ cup chicken broth
2 tablespoons butter
Salt and pepper to taste
4 ounces sharp cheese
¼ cup heavy cream

Directions:
1. Add all of the ingredients into the Crock Pot.
2. Close the lid. Set the pot on High and cook for 3 hours.
3. Blend with an immersion blender until smooth.
4. Serve warm.

Nutritional Information (Per Serving)
Calories: 148; Fat: 11 g; Net Carbohydrates: 4.3 g; Protein: 6 g

Broccoli Cauliflower "Rice"

Serves: 8
Cooking Time: 2–3 hours
Ingredients:
1 pound cauliflower, grated
8 ounces broccoli, chopped
4–5 tablespoons water
4 tablespoons butter
1 tablespoon lemon zest, grated
2 cloves garlic, minced
½ teaspoon garlic salt or salt
¼ cup Parmesan cheese, grated
Pepper to taste
1 medium onion, minced

Directions:
1. Add cauliflower and broccoli into the Crock Pot. Sprinkle water over it.

2. Close the lid. Set the pot on High and cook for about 2–3 hours.

3. Add rest of the ingredients and stir. Cover and set aside for a while for the flavors to set in.

4. Serve warm.

Nutritional Information (Per Serving)
Calories: 91; Fat: 8.5 g: Net Carbohydrates: 4 g; Protein: 3 g

Italian Zucchini and Yellow Squash

Serves: 3
Cooking Time: 5–6 hours
Ingredients:
1 medium yellow squash, quartered, sliced
1 medium zucchini, quartered, sliced
1 teaspoon Italian seasoning or to taste
¼ teaspoon sea salt
2 tablespoons Parmesan cheese, grated
Pepper to taste
½ teaspoon garlic powder
2 tablespoons cold butter, cubed

Directions:
1. Add squash and zucchini into the Crock Pot.
2. Sprinkle with salt, garlic powder, pepper, and Italian seasoning.
3. Place butter cubes all over the vegetables. Sprinkle cheese on top.
4. Close the lid. Set the pot on Low and cook for 5–6 hours or until tender.
5. Stir and serve.

Nutritional Information (Per Serving)
Calories: 122; Fat: 9.9 g; Net Carbohydrates: 5.4 g; Protein: 4.2 g

Coconut Creamed Spinach

Serves: 4
Cooking Time: 2–3 hours
Ingredients:
½ cup coconut milk
¼ teaspoon ground nutmeg
¼ teaspoon cayenne pepper
8 cups baby spinach
4 teaspoons swerve
Salt to taste

Directions:
1. Add all the ingredients into the Crock Pot.
2. Close the lid. Set the pot on Low and cook for 2–3 hours.
3. Stir and serve.

Nutritional Information (Per Serving)
Calories: 84; Fat: 7.5 g; Net Carbohydrates: 7 g; Protein: 2.4 g

Garlic Mushrooms

Serves: 3
Cooking Time: 3 hours
Ingredients:
1 pound white button mushrooms, quartered
3 garlic cloves, minced
¼ cup fresh parsley, chopped
½ cup vegetable broth
Salt and pepper to taste
2 tablespoons butter, melted
1 teaspoon fresh lemon zest, grated finely

Directions:
1. In a Crock Pot, add all ingredients except lemon zest and butter, and mix well.
2. Set the pot on High. Cover and cook for 2–3 hours.
3. Uncover the Crock Pot, and drizzle with the melted butter.
4. Serve with a topping of lemon zest.

Nutritional Information (Per Serving)
Calories: 107; Fat: 8.2 g; Net Carbohydrates: 4.6 g; Protein: 5.2 g

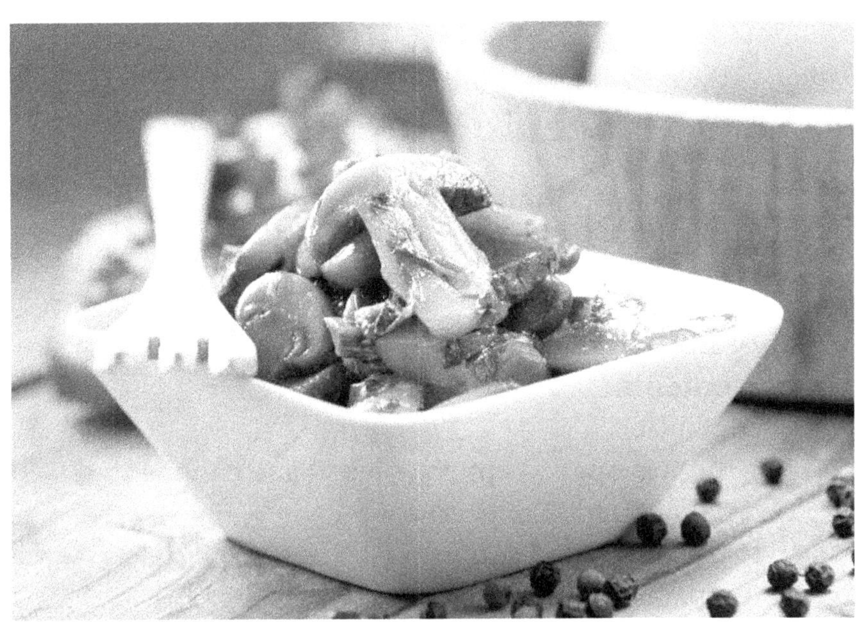

CHAPTER EIGHT

Ketogenic Soup Recipes

Creamy and Cheesy Soup

Serves: 6
Cooking Time: 6 hours
Ingredients:
¼ cup butter
4 medium jalapeño peppers, seeded and chopped
1 teaspoon dried thyme, crushed
½ teaspoon ground cumin
½ teaspoon ground coriander
3½ cups chicken broth
8 ounces cheddar cheese, shredded
¾ cup heavy cream
Salt and pepper to taste
2 bacon slices, cooked and chopped

Directions:

1. In a soup pan, melt butter over medium heat. Add jalapeño peppers, and sauté for about 1–2 minutes. Transfer to the Crock Pot.

2. Add the herbs and chicken broth, and stir.

3. Close the lid. Set the pot on Low and cook for 6 hours.

4. Blend with an immersion blender until smooth.

5. Stir in cheddar cheese, heavy cream, salt, and pepper. Cover and cook on High for 20-30 minutes.

6. Serve hot with a topping of bacon.

Nutritional Information (Per Serving)
Calories: 410; Fat: 32.1 g; Net Carbohydrates: 3.8 g; Protein: 24.8 g

Pizza Soup

Serves: 4
Cooking Time: 6–7 hours
Ingredients:
½ pound Italian sausage
8 ounces canned crushed tomatoes
1 can (16 ounces) mushrooms or equal amount of fresh mushrooms
1 small onion, chopped
¼ pound pepperoni, thinly sliced
1 teaspoon dried oregano
1 cup beef broth
1 small green pepper, chopped
½ teaspoon garlic powder
1 teaspoon Italian seasoning
½ cup mozzarella cheese, freshly grated
2 tablespoons Parmesan cheese, grated

Directions:
1. Place a skillet with sausage over medium heat. Cook until brown. Drain excess fat and transfer sausage into the Crock Pot.

2. Add rest of the ingredients except both cheese and stir.

3. Close the lid. Set the pot on Low and cook for 6–7 hours.

4. Ladle into soup bowls. Garnish with both the cheese and serve.

Nutritional Information (Per Serving)
Calories: 449; Fat: 32.7 g; Carbohydrate: 12.7 g; Protein: 27.5 g

Cabbage Roll Soup

Serves: 6
Cooking Time: 3 hours
Ingredients:
2 tablespoons olive oil
¼ cup onion, chopped
2 shallots, chopped
1¼ pounds ground beef
½ teaspoon salt
2 cloves garlic, minced
½ teaspoon dried oregano
½ teaspoon dried parsley
½ teaspoon pepper powder
12 ounces keto friendly marinara sauce
1 cup cauliflower, grated to rice like texture
3 cups beef broth
6 cups cabbage, thinly sliced

Directions:
1. Add oil into a saucepan and place over medium heat.
2. Add onions and shallots and sauté until translucent.
3. Stir in ground beef. Sauté until it is brown. Add spices, salt, and dried herbs. Sauté for a few seconds until fragrant. Transfer into the Crock Pot.
4. Add marinara sauce and mix well. Add cauliflower and stir until well combined.
5. Add beef broth and cabbage and stir well.
6. Close the lid. Set the pot on High and cook for 3 hours
7. Ladle into soup bowls and serve.

Nutritional Information (Per Serving)
Calories: 361; Fat: 28.8 g; Net Carbohydrates: 4.3 g; Protein: 18.8 g

Low Carb Chicken Noodle Soup

Serves: 6
Cooking Time: 6 hours
Ingredients:
3 tablespoons coconut oil
1½ cups celery, chopped
9 green onions, green parts, only, chopped
1½ pounds chicken thighs, skinless, boneless
9 cups chicken stock
¾ teaspoon dried oregano
1 teaspoon dried basil
1½ teaspoons salt
3 cups spiralized daikon noodles
Freshly ground pepper to taste

Directions:
1. Using a spiralizer make noodles of the daikon. Use 3 cups of the daikon noodles.

2. Place a skillet with oil over medium heat. Add chicken and cook until brown on both the sides. Transfer into the Crock Pot.

3. Add rest of the ingredients except daikon noodles and stir.

4. Close the lid. Set the pot on Low and cook for 6 hours.

5. When done, remove chicken with a slotted spoon and place on your work area. When cool enough to handle, shred the chicken with a pair of forks and add it back into the pot. Stir and heat thoroughly.

6. Add noodles and stir.

7. Ladle into soup bowls and serve.

Nutritional Information (Per Serving)
Calories: 226; Fat: 12.4 g; Net Carbohydrates: 3.5 g, Protein: 24.1 g

Taco Soup

Serves: 4
Cooking Time: 6 hours
Ingredients:
1 pound ground beef
1 tablespoon butter, melt
1 tablespoon taco seasoning
10 ounces canned diced tomatoes
8 ounces cream cheese
2 cups chicken broth
Salt and pepper to taste
¼ cup Cheddar cheese, shredded to garnish
Cilantro to garnish

Directions:
1. Place a skillet with butter and beef over medium heat. Cook until brown and transfer into the Crock Pot.

2. Add rest of the ingredients except Cheddar and cilantro, and mix well.

3. Close the lid. Set the pot on Low and cook for 6 hours.

4. Ladle into soup bowls and serve garnished with Cheddar and cilantro.

Nutritional Information (Per Serving)
Calories: 628; Fat: 53.8 g; Net Carbohydrates: 6.9 g; Protein: 27.1 g

Kale Chicken Soup

Serves: 4
Cooking Time: 6 hours
Ingredients:
1 pound chicken thighs
1 spring fresh thyme
1 tablespoon fresh thyme, chopped
Salt and pepper to taste
1 clove garlic, minced
2½ cups chicken broth
2 tablespoons olive oil
1 medium onion, chopped
2 cups packed kale, discard hard stems and ribs, chopped

Directions:
1. Sprinkle salt and pepper over the chicken and place in the Crock Pot.
2. Sprinkle garlic over the chicken. Add water, chicken broth, oil and thyme sprig and stir.
3. Close the lid. Set the pot on High and cook for 4 hours. Remove the chicken with a slotted spoon and place on your cutting board. When cool enough to handle, shred with a pair of forks. Discard the thyme.
4. Add the bones back into the Crock Pot. Refrigerate the chicken.
5. Add rest of the ingredients.
6. Cover and cook on High for 2 hours.
7. Discard the bones and add chicken into the pot during the last 10 minutes of cooking.
8. Ladle into soup bowls and serve.

Nutritional Information (Per Serving)
Calories: 411; Fat: 26.7 g; Net Carbohydrates: 7.8 g; Protein: 33.1 g

Cauliflower and Ham Soup

Serves: 5
Cooking Time: 2½ hours
Ingredients:
12 ounces cauliflower florets
1 cup water
3 cups chicken broth
½ teaspoon onion powder
¼ teaspoon garlic powder
1½ cups ham, chopped
2 teaspoons fresh thyme leaves, chopped
1 tablespoon apple cider vinegar
1 tablespoon butter
Salt and pepper to taste

Directions:
1. Add cauliflower, onion powder, garlic powder, water, and broth into the Crock Pot.

2. Close the lid. Set the pot on Low and cook for 4 hours or until cauliflower is soft.

3. Blend with an immersion blender until smooth.

4. Add ham and thyme leaves. Cover and cook on High for 30 minutes.

5. Add butter, salt, pepper, and apple cider vinegar and stir.

6. Ladle into soup bowls and serve.

Nutritional Information (Per Serving)
Calories: 305; Fat: 16 g; Net Carbohydrates: 6.6 g; Protein: 29 g

Jalapeño Popper Soup

Serves: 4
Cooking Time: 3 hours
Ingredients:
1½ tablespoons butter
1 small onion, chopped
1–2 jalapeños, deseed if desired, chopped
½ small green pepper, chopped
Salt and pepper to taste
¾ pound chicken breast, skinless, boneless
1½ cups chicken broth
1 large clove garlic, minced
¼ pound bacon, cooked until crisp, crumbled
¼ teaspoon paprika
¼ teaspoon xanthan gum
6 tablespoons cheddar cheese, shredded
6 tablespoons Monterrey Jack cheese, shredded
3 ounces cream cheese
¼ cup heavy whipping cream
½ teaspoon ground cumin

Directions:
1. Place a saucepan with butter over medium heat. Add onion, jalapeño, green pepper, salt, and pepper. Sauté for 2–3 minutes and transfer into the Crock Pot.
2. Add chicken and broth.
3. Close the lid. Set the pot on High and cook for 3 hours.
4. When done, remove chicken with a slotted spoon and place on your cutting board. Shred chicken with a fork and add it back into the pot.
5. Add rest of the ingredients and stir until cheese melts.
6. Ladle into soup bowls and serve.

CHAPTER NINE

Ketogenic Snack Recipes

Cheesy Spinach Artichoke Dip

Serves: 14
Cooking Time: 2 hours
Ingredients:
2 cans (14 ounces each) artichoke hearts, drained, finely chopped
20 ounces baby spinach
2 cups mozzarella cheese, grated
16 ounces cream cheese
½ cup milk
2/3 cup Parmesan cheese, grated
4 teaspoons minced garlic
¼ teaspoon cayenne pepper
Salt and pepper to taste

Directions:
1. Add all ingredients into the Crock Pot and stir.
2. Close the lid, set the pot on High, and cook for 2 hours.
3. Stir and serve with vegetable sticks.

Nutritional Information (Per Serving)
Calories: 179; Fat: 13.4 g; Net Carbohydrates: 4.9 g; Protein: 8.4 g

Buffalo Chicken Dip

Serves: 4
Cooking Time: 1½ hours
Ingredients:
4 ounces cream cheese, softened, cubed
1 cup mozzarella cheese, shredded
2 ounces blue cheese, crumbled
1½ cups deli rotisserie chicken, diced
½ cup sour cream
½ tablespoon Ranch seasoning
2 tablespoons jalapeños (optional), to top
2 green onions, thinly sliced + extra to garnish
½ cup hot sauce + extra to serve

Directions:
1. Spray the inside of the Crock Pot with cooking spray.

2. Add all the ingredients into the Crock Pot and mix well.

3. Close the lid. Set the pot on High and cook for 1½ hours.

4. Serve warm garnished with jalapeños, hot sauce and green onions.

5. Serve with celery sticks or keto crackers.

Nutritional Information (Per Serving)
Calories: 347; Fat: 28 g; Net Carbohydrates: 2.4 g; Protein: 20 g

Meatballs

Serves: 12
Cooking Time: 2 hours
Ingredients:
8 ounces ground beef chuck
2 ounces mozzarella cheese
1 small egg
2 ounce hard Parmesan cheese, grated
3 cloves garlic, minced

Directions:
1. Mix together all the ingredients in a bowl.
2. Divide into 12 equal portions and shape into balls.
3. Place in the Crock Pot that is lined with foil. Close the lid, set the pot on High and cook for 2 hours or until done.
4. Insert toothpicks and serve.

Nutritional Information (Per Serving, 1 meatball)
Calories: 78.8; Fat: 5.8 g; Net Carbohydrates: 0.5 g; Protein: 6.1 g

Lemon Garlic Chicken Kebabs

Serves: 2
Cooking Time: 3-4 hours
Ingredients:

¾ pound chicken thighs, skinless, boneless, cut into 2 inch pieces

1 tablespoon lemon juice

1 tablespoon garlic, minced

½ teaspoon salt

2 tablespoons fresh lemon juice

½ teaspoon dried oregano

3 tablespoons olive oil

4 bamboo skewers

Directions:

1. Add all the cooking ingredients except chicken into a zip lock bag and shake well.

2. Add chicken and shake well. Let it marinate for 60–90 minutes.

3. Trim the bamboo skewers to fit into your Crock Pot. Thread the chicken on to the skewers.

4. Place in the Crock Pot. Cover, set the pot on High and cook for 3–4 hours. Check after 3 hours of cooking.

Nutritional Information (Per Serving)
Calories: 260; Fat: 12.9 g; Net Carbohydrates: 1 g; Protein: 34 g

Buffalo Chicken Wings

Serves: 8
Cooking Time: 5 hours
Ingredients:
1½ pounds chicken wings
1 tablespoon butter, melted
⅓ cup Ranch dressing
12 ounces chicken wing sauce
1 teaspoon hot sauce or to taste

Directions:
1. Add butter, chicken wing sauce and hot sauce into the Crock Pot and mix well.
2. Add chicken wings and stir until is well coated.
3. Close the lid. Set the pot on Low and cook for 4–5 hours or on High for 2–2½ hours.
4. Serve hot or warm with blue cheese dressing.

Nutritional Information (Per Serving)
Calories: 213; Fat: 15 g; Net Carbohydrates: 2.6 g; Protein: 15.9 g

CHAPTER TEN

Ketogenic Dessert Recipes

Pumpkin Custard

Serves: 6
Cooking Time: 3 hours
Ingredients:
15 ounces pumpkin puree
4 eggs, beaten
½ cup heavy cream
2 teaspoons pumpkin pie spice
2 teaspoons vanilla extract
½ teaspoon liquid stevia
½ teaspoon salt
⅓ cup whipped cream

Directions:
1. Grease 6 ramekins.
2. In a large bowl, add all ingredients except whipped cream, and beat until smooth.
3. Divide mixture evenly in prepared ramekins. Cover them with foil.
4. Pour about 2 cups water into the Crock Pot. Place a rack in it. Place the ramekins on the rack.
5. Close the lid. Set the pot on High and cook for 3 hours, or until set.
6. Remove the ramekins from the pot, and place on a wire rack to cool.
7. Serve warm or cold with a topping of whipped cream.

Blackberry Pudding

Serves: 4
Cooking Time: 3 hours
Ingredients:
For dry ingredients:
½ cup coconut flour
½ teaspoon baking powder

For wet ingredients:
10 large egg yolks
4 tablespoons butter, melted
4 teaspoons lemon juice
½ cup blackberries
20 drops liquid stevia
4 tablespoons coconut oil, melted
4 tablespoons heavy cream
Zest of 2 lemons, grated
4 tablespoons erythritol

Directions:
1. Mix together the dry ingredients in a bowl.
2. Add butter and coconut oil into a 2nd bowl and mix well.
3. Add yolks into a 3rd bowl and beat until they turn pale yellow in color. Add stevia and beat until combined.
4. Add cream, lemon juice and lemon zest into the 2nd bowl. Beat until well combined. Add the egg yolk mixture and beat again.
5. Add the dry ingredients into the 2nd bowl and mix until well combined.

6. Grease 4 ramekins and divide the batter among the ramekins. Place blackberries on top. Push it lightly into the batter.

7. Place the ramekins in the Crock Pot. Pour enough water around the ramekins to reach up to half the ramekins.

8. Close the lid. Set the pot on High and cook for 3 hours.

9. When done, cool completely and place in the refrigerator for a few hours to chill.

10. Run a knife around the edges of the ramekins. Invert on to a plate.

11. You can also serve warm.

Nutritional Information (Per Serving)
Calories: 478; Fat: 43.5 g; Net Carbohydrates: 10.7 g; Protein: 9 g

Keto Brownies

Makes: 32 pieces
Cooking Time: 2–3 hours
Ingredients:
10 ounces low carb milk chocolate, melted
6 large eggs
½ cup mascarpone cheese
1 teaspoon salt
8 tablespoons butter, melted
1 cup swerve
½ cup cocoa powder, unsweetened

Directions:
1. Grease the inside of the Crock Pot generously with butter.

2. Whisk together the butter and chocolate in a bowl.

3. Add eggs and sweetener into another bowl and beat with an electric mixer until pale in color.

4. Beat in the mascarpone cheese. Add a little cocoa and salt at a time into the bowl of eggs and beat well each time.

5. Add chocolate mixture and fold gently.

6. Pour into the Crock Pot.

7. Close the lid. Set the pot on High and cook for 2–3 hours or until a toothpick inserted in the center of the cake comes out clean.

8. Cool for a while and slice into 32 equal pieces.

9. Serve warm or at room temperature.

Nutritional Information (Per Brownie)
Calories: 86.9; Fat: 8 g; Net Carbohydrates: 5.3 g; Protein: 2.2 g

Dark Chocolate Cake

Serves: 5
Cooking Time: 2–3 hours
Ingredients:
3 tablespoons sugar free chocolate chips

For dry ingredients:
½ cup + 1 tablespoon almond flour
¼ cup cocoa powder, unsweetened
¾ teaspoon baking powder
¼ cup swerve
1½ tablespoons unflavored whey protein powder
A large pinch salt

For wet ingredients:
3 small eggs
⅓ cup almond milk, unsweetened
3 tablespoons butter, melted
½ teaspoon vanilla extract

Directions:
1. Grease the inside of the Crock Pot generously with butter.

2. Add all the dry ingredients into a bowl. Mix well.

3. Add all the wet ingredients into another bowl. Beat to mix well. Add chocolate chips and stir.

4. Add dry ingredients into the bowl of wet ingredients and mix until a batter is formed.

5. Pour the batter into the Crock Pot.

6. Close the lid. Set the pot on High and cook for 2–3 hours or until a toothpick inserted in the center of the cake comes out clean.

7. Serve warm with whipped cream.

Mocha Walnut Coffee Cups

Serves: 6
Cooking Time: 45–60 minutes
Ingredients:
¼ cup coconut oil
½ cup cocoa powder, unsweetened
1½ packets stevia or to taste
2 tablespoons walnut butter
1 tablespoon sugar free coffee liqueur syrup
2 tablespoons heavy whipping cream
12 walnuts halves

Directions:
1. Add all the ingredients except cream and walnuts into the Crock Pot.
2. Close the lid. Set the pot on Hight and cook for 45–60 minutes until melted.
3. Add cream and mix until well combined.
4. Take a 12-count mini muffin cup mold and divide the mixture into it.
5. Place a walnut piece in each cup. Freeze until set.
6. Remove from the mold and transfer into an airtight container. Refrigerate until serving.

Lemon Custard

Serves: 8
Cooking Time: 3 hours
Ingredients:
10 large egg yolks
2 tablespoons lemon zest
1 teaspoon liquid stevia
½ cup fresh lemon juice
2 teaspoons vanilla extract
4 cups heavy cream
Whipped cream, lightly sweetened with stevia

Directions:
1. Add yolks, vanilla, stevia, lemon juice and zest into a bowl and whisk well. Add heavy cream and whisk well. Pour into 8 ramekins. Cover them with foil.

2. Pour about 2 cups water into the Crock Pot. Place a rack in it. Place the ramekins on the rack.

3. Close the lid. Set the pot on High and cook for 3 hours, or until set.

4. When done, cool completely and place the ramekins in the refrigerator for a few hours to chill.

5. Spoon whipped cream on top and serve.

Nutritional Information (Per Serving, without whipped cream)
Calories: 319; Fat: 30 g; Net Carbohydrates: 2.9 g; Protein: 7 g

Conclusion

If you want to lose weight the healthier way, the ketogenic diet is for you. I hope the delicious Crock Pot recipes in this book will help you kick-start the ketogenic lifestyle and enjoy its various health benefits.

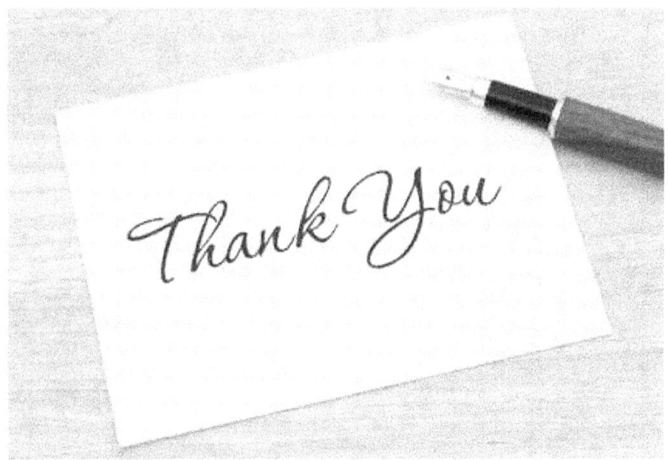

Finally, I want to thank you for reading my book. If you enjoyed the book, please share your thoughts and post a review on the book retailer's website. It would be greatly appreciated!

Best wishes,

Jasmine King

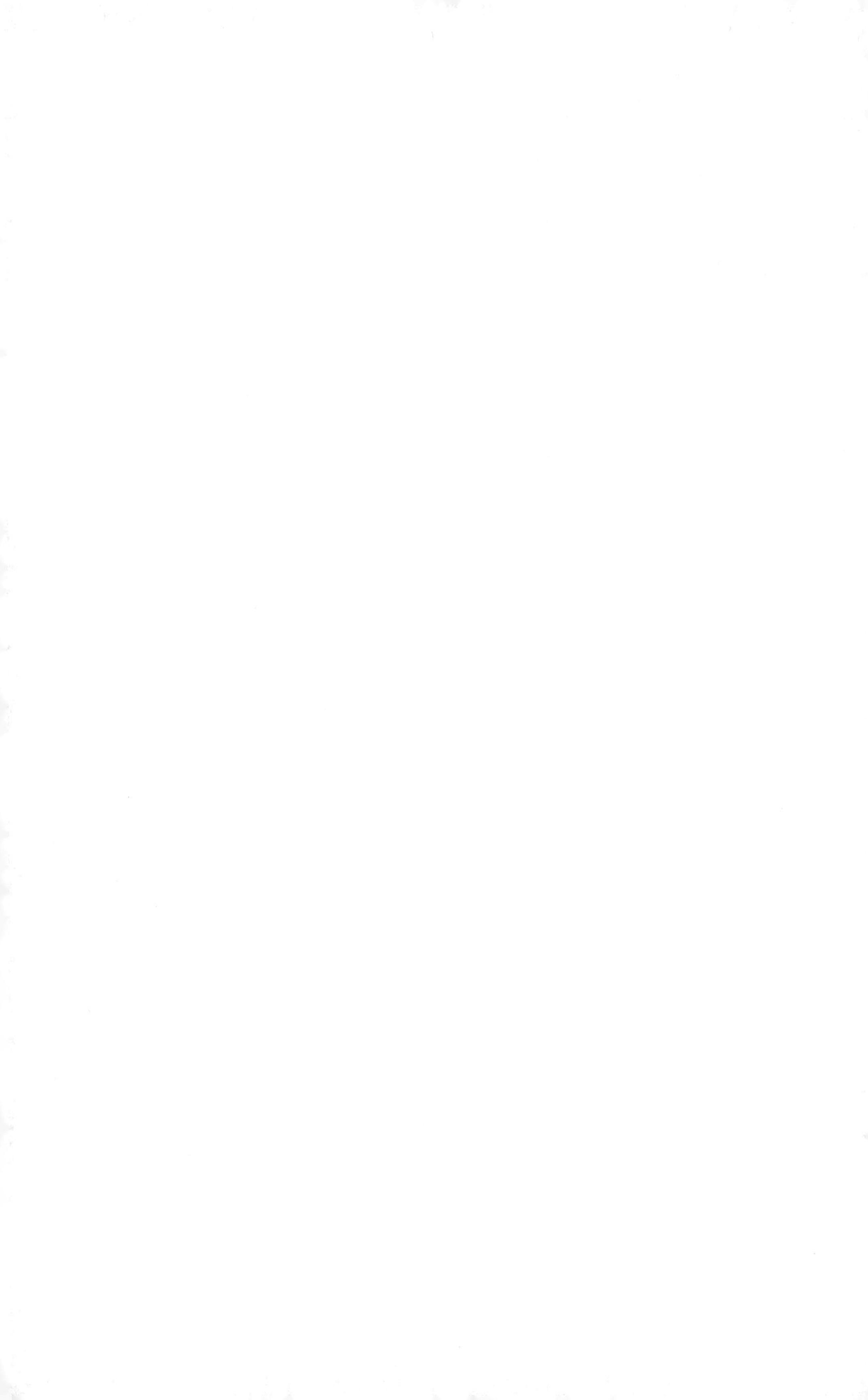